CHAPTER 1

Introduction

KU-186-634

HISTORY OF ANTENATAL INVESTIGATIONS

Historically, antenatal care is a recent phenomenon. McIntyre, a doctor practicing in Scotland in the early 1900s is credited with being the 'father of antenatal care', but his involvement only went as far as the recognition that disadvantaged women had better outcomes in childbirth if they were allowed some rest and had reasonable nutrition in the antenatal period.

The idea that tests and interventions could improve the success rate of pregnancies was still in its infancy. Although the former Central Midwives Board did stipulate that midwives should "enquire into" a pregnant woman's health, by the 1930s there is evidence that this was still not being followed with any regularity (Young, 1987).

The first antenatal test that could be carried out and identified with some accuracy was urine testing, although it involved a complicated procedure. Proteinuria could be diagnosed, and it was recognised that this was a pathological sign, but there was no treatment to offer other than rest, a milk diet and purgatives! (Berkeley, 1924)

Today the investigations that can be done in the antenatal period are many, varied and are becoming extremely complex. The field has expanded rapidly and is changing almost daily as research findings question the value of some established tests, (such as regularly recording the weight of women within the normal weight/height range), and advances in medical science are applied to practice, for example genetic typing (Weatherall, 1991).

PROVISION OF ANTENATAL INVESTIGATIONS

Not every area can afford to routinely offer all women the full range of antenatal tests available, but this does not necessarily mean that women are being deprived of essential care. As investigations and subsequent care become more sophisticated, centres of specialisation with highly trained personnel and complex equipment are being established. The role of those working outside these centres is to be aware of the latest developments, and to offer the appropriate screening tests to those women who would benefit from referral for more intensive investigations.

Tests offered need to be cost effective. These days limited resources mean that routinely carrying out expensive tests on inappropriate clients costs money that could, perhaps, be used more productively elsewhere. Many conditions are more common in one geographical area than in another: for example, neural tube defects occur more often in Scotland and Wales than in England. For this reason, each centre needs to look carefully at its population to ensure the investigations offered reflect their clients' needs.

RESULTS OF INVESTIGATIONS

How women receive the results of their investigations can be a vital part of their antenatal care. For some women, to be told over the telephone that their haemoglobin level is low, or that they have a urinary tract infection, is perfectly acceptable. Others may perceive this as devastating news. As these conditions should be treated as soon as possible, it is not appropriate to wait for the next routine antenatal visit, and yet sending a woman a non-informative letter asking her merely to "attend her antenatal clinic or general practitioner's surgery as soon as possible" may be even more disturbing than hearing exactly what is wrong.

It is obviously not cost effective to employ midwives to visit all women individually with each minor abnormal result. The answer is probably to ensure that every woman who has any test performed knows why it is being done, and exactly what a normal or abnormal result will mean. This may be a time consuming exercise, but it is one that should increase a woman's satisfaction with her antenatal care.

There are many aspects concerned with the giving of investigation results, whether minor or major, positive or negative, which should be well known to all midwives. The environment in which the result is given is important - the staff should be unrushed, and privacy ensured. Ideally the person giving the results should be known to the woman, and someone whom she trusts enough to question. The woman should have a way of contacting the midwife after her visit, in case questions occur to her later.

Confidentiality needs to be ensured at all times, concerning all tests, no matter how trivial. A woman who feels any infection is 'dirty' and a reflection on her will not appreciate having the news of her urinary tract infection broadcast to the waiting room at large.

Giving results of tests which have, potentially,a life-threatening implication, such as amniocentisis or HIV investigation, means that sensitivity and skilled communication need to be considered. This will become an even more common aspect of antenatal care as more and more tests to determine the health of the fetus are developed. The provision of two-tiered result giving (i.e. negative results are given over the phone, whereas those with positive results are asked to attend clinic) soon becomes known throughout the community. Being given an appointment to obtain the outcome is tantamount to saying there is a positive result.

Many centres ask both parents to attend when results of amniocentesis are given, or arrange for a community midwife to visit women at home to give the results. All systems will have drawbacks for some couples. When giving life-changing information the way in which test results are divulged needs to be carefully considered, with regard to clients' needs and local resources.

Follow up counselling is necessary for very many investigations, even if the result is negative. Those whose amniocentesis result is normal need to be aware that this result is no guarantee of a baby free of any defects. Those with a negative HIV result may need further information about safe sex and risk behaviours.

Therefore, counselling can be seen as a vital part of many investigations, as part of the health education role of the midwife. To this end each midwife needs to ensure her counselling skills are up to date and used appropriately.

References: CHAPTER 1

Berkeley C A Handbook of Midwifery 1924 Cassell & Co. Ltd. London.

Weatherall D J The New Genetics and Clinical PracticeThird Edition 1991 Oxford University Press, Oxford.

Young P "Yesterday's District Midwife" Midwives Chronicle & Nursing Notes June 1987 pp.173-175.

CHAPTER 2

Preconception Care

The value of carrying out preconception investigations, and treating any deficiencies to ensure a couple is in optimum health at the moment of conception, is stated widely. However, current research seems to be suggesting that many pre-pregnancy interventions are of unproven benefit (Lumley & Astbury, 1989; Lancet 1985). In fact provision of this service by the National Health Service(NHS) is practically non-existent, although there are private agencies who will screen and advise those seeking to become pregnant. Many NHS hospitals and general practitioners' surgeries have specialised clinics (for example 'recurrent miscarriage clinics' or 'diabetic clinics') where preconception advice is available to those attending. The majority of couples however, have no preconception resources available to them, other than self-help publications.

There can be no doubt that those suffering from a medical condition, such as anaemia, hypertension or an infection, should seek medical treatment before undertaking pregnancy. However despite recent scientific advances, we still have no clear knowledge of how to avoid premature delivery, poor fetal growth or many congenital birth defects. While claims for detailed nutritional/chemical analyses purport to explain these poor outcomes, there are few studies to back up such assertions. One of the exceptions to this is the work which shows a link between maternal folate deficiency and neural tube defects (Rosenberg, 1992). Based on the now seemingly conclusive evidence, recommendations are being made to all women planning to become pregnant to increase their dietary folate intake and to take a folic acid supplement (0.4mg) daily (Department of Health, 1992). Those who have had a previous pregnancy complicated with this condition are recommended to take increased supplements.

There are also other studies that suggest vitamins may have a role to play in avoiding congenital malformations (Department of Health, 1992).

Basic good health measures such as stopping smoking, limiting (or stopping) consumption of alcohol, regular exercise and good dietary habits will bring undoubted benefits to the potential parents. Midwives should always remember that their role encompasses health education.

This chapter contains some of the tests that can be done in the pre-pregnancy period.

BLOOD GROUP

Blood is typed as A, B, AB or O depending on the presence or absence of specific agglutinogens on the erythrocytes. The Rhesus factor is added to identify the blood group as either negative or positive depending on whether the Rhesus antigen is present. It is valuable for all individuals to know their blood group, but for a woman planning pregnancy it is particularly important because of the risk of haemorrhage or shock during pregnancy or childbirth. Blood can then be X-matched more quickly for transfusion. The Rhesus factor and antibody status are also identified because, if the woman is Rhesus negative, further tests will be required.

Antibodies

Certain antibodies can be present in a woman's blood, which could influence the health of her baby, as well as cause a reaction to a blood transfusion.

ABO and Rhesus are the most common antibodies which can cause haemolytic disease in the newborn. Other less common antibodies which can cause the same effect include Kell, Duffy and Kidd (Hoffbrand & Pettit, 1993).

If those antibodies that are potentially dangerous to the fetus are identified early, there are now treatments available, such as fetal blood transfusion, which could possibly maintain a healthy fetus. Monitoring antibody levels during the pregnancy could ensure delivery at the optimum time.

Rhesus (Rh) Factor

Rhesus blood group factors are inherited and the C,D and E genes are dominant, D being most common. About 85% of Caucasian, and 99% of other races, are Rhesus positive. An individual is considered Rhesus positive if she possesses a D factor.

If the D factor is introduced to a Rhesus negative woman, for example by blood transfusion or transplacentally during pregnancy (whether carried to term or not), she will produce antibodies against it.

The transfer of maternal antibodies to the Rhesus positive fetus will cause haemolysis (destruction of red blood cells). The degree of haemolysis will determine the severity of the effect on the fetus, which could range from mild anaemia to hydrops fetalis. (See Chapter 7 for details of Rhesus isoimmunisation.)

Full Blood Count

The normal values for non-pregnant females are:-

Hb (Haemoglobin)	11.5 to 15.5 g/dl
RBC (Red Blood Cells/Erythrocytes)	3.5 to 5.6 x 10^{12}/1
PCV (Packed Cell Volume/Haematocrit)	36 - 48%
MCV (Mean Cell Volume)	76 - 96 fl
MCH (Mean Cell Haemoglobin)	27 - 34 µg
MCHC (Mean Cell Haemoglobin Concentration)	20 35 g/dl
WCC (Whie Cell Count/Leucocytes)	4.0 - 11.0 x 10^9/1
Platelets	150 - 400 x 10^9/1

Table 1: Normal Blood Values

Haemoglobinopathies

Haemoglobinopathy is an inherited abnormality of haemoglobin in the red blood cells. This results in either early haemolysis of the red blood cells or decreased production of haemoglobin. The most common haemoglobinopathies are sickle cell disease and thalassaemia.

See Chapter 7 for details of diagnosis in pregnancy.

Sickle Cell

This is seen mainly in those of African, Caribbean, Mediterranean, Middle Eastern or Asian Indian origin. As the condition is recessive, only those inheriting the Hb-S gene from both parents will have Sickle Cell Disease. Hb-CC (homozygous CC disease) is not a sickling disorder because there is no S gene. If a woman is carrying only one Hb-S or Hb-C gene (sickle cell trait) or has Sickle Cell Disease (Hb-SS) herself, it is necessary to test her partner In this way, a prediction can be made of the risk of her baby either having the disease or being a carrier.

a)

| | | **Mother** (sickle cell trait) | |
		X	S
Father	X	XX	XS
(sickle cell trait)	S	XS	XS

Offspring: 25% chance of being normal; 25% chance of having sickle cell anaemia; 50% chance of sickle cell trait

b)

| | | **Mother** (sickle cell trait) | |
		X	S
Father	S	XS	SS
(sickle cell anaemia)	S	XS	SS

Offspring: 50% chance of having sickle cell anaemia or sickle cell trait.

c)

| | | **Mother** (normal) | |
		X	X
Father	X	X	XX
(sickle cell trait)	S	XS	XX

Offspring: 50% chance of being normal or having sickle cell trait.

Table 2: Examples of inheritance of sickle cell disease.
S, gene for HB-S; X, gene for normal haemoglobin

To test for the presence of HbS, red blood cells are observed for sickling when exposed to very low oxygen tensions, or a sickle solubility (Sickledex) test is carried out. If HbS is identified then electrophoresis is carried out to detect any variation, in particular HbSC. HbSC (heterozygous sickle cell haemoglobin C disease) is much milder than HbSS and usually causes few problems, but during pregnancy or the puerperium the HbSC woman can sometimes have an unexpected serious (or even fatal) sickling crisis.

Thalassaemia

Thalassaemia is a condition affecting the globin chain, with either alpha or beta chains missing. There are four alpha chains, and if all four are missing (alpha thalassaemia major) this is incompatible with life. Beta thalassaemia major is a life-threatening disease, requiring treatment such as frequent blood transfusions and regular drug therapy for survival, but those with thalassaemia minor have few, if any, symptoms.

Thalassaemia is seen mainly in those of Mediterranean, Middle Eastern or South East Asian origin. Beta thalassaemia is particularly common in those from Cyprus, Sardinia and parts of Italy and Greece.

Like sickle cell disease, this condition is also recessive. Those women who carry a thalassaemia trait (thalassaemia minor) need to have the results of their partner's test before a prediction about the baby's condition can be made.

Blood results in thalassaemia show the haemoglobin, the Mean Cell Volume (MCV) and the Mean Cell Haemoglobin (MCH) are reduced, but the serum iron can be raised. Electrophoresis will usually confirm the condition, but an alpha chain count will be necessary if alpha thalassaemia trait is suspected.

Hepatitis B

Screening for Hepatitis B in pregnancy is routinely carried out in many antenatal clinics. A susceptible woman, especially one whose work, or life-style, puts her at risk (for example, she has regular contact with blood or blood products), may wish to be vaccinated prior to pregnancy. The vaccination is given in three parts, with the second part one month after the first and the last five months later. Serum is then tested after two months for immunity levels. There is no known teratogenic effect on the fetus if pregnancy occurs during the course of treatment. (See Chapter 8 for Hepatitis B in pregnancy.)

Human Immunodeficiency Virus (HIV)

Some women will wish to have their HIV status checked before undertaking a pregnancy, and it can be argued that this is a far better time than in the antenatal period. This way, if the result is positive, the extreme trauma will not be exacerbated by the limited time available to consider decisions concerning her pregnancy. (See Chapter 8 for details of HIV in pregnancy.)

Rubella

Since 1970 schoolgirls in the UK between the ages of 11 and 14 have been vaccinated against rubella. In 1981 the age for vaccination was reduced to 10 years and efforts have been made to increase the uptake of rubella vaccination. However, some women who have been vaccinated, show an unprotective level of immunity during routine screening in pregnancy. It is recommended that all women planning a pregnancy have their rubella status checked and a further vaccination if necessary. Following vaccination, it is strongly advised that pregnancy is avoided for three months, as rubella is a live vaccine and therefore may have a teratogenic effect on the fetus. (See Chapter 8 for details of diagnosis in pregnancy.)

Syphilis

A test for syphylis is routinely carried out in the antenatal period, but if done before conception any necessary treatment can be completed before pregnancy commences. (See Chapter 8 for details of syphilis in pregnancy.)

Cervical Smear

The Royal College of Obstetricians and Gynaecologists recommend that all women who are sexually active or over 25 years old should have cervical smears every 3 years. If a woman is due for a smear, this could be carried out in the preconception period rather in pregnancy. (See Chapter 12 for a description of smear results.)

Urine Tests

Urine may be tested for infection as women can have asymptomatic bacteriuria. As this may have a harmful effect in pregnancy, causing a renal infection which could lead to premature labour, treating it before conception would be sensible.

Glucose present in the urine before pregnancy could indicate diabetes mellitus, and further investigations, such as a glucose tolerance test, would be necessary.

Hair Analysis

It is possible to use cells of hair follicles to test for such metabolic disorders as Hunter's syndrome (a rare autosomal X-linked recessive condition which includes mental retardation and deafness), but this is an expensive procedure, and is not commonly done. Private hair analysis can be undertaken to produce an evaluation of essential mineral levels, and to diagnose toxic metal levels.

Counselling

Specific preconception counselling, and tests, may be appropriate for some women. Those who have had a previous ectopic pregnancy are recommended to attend for an early (6 week) ultrasound scan as soon as they suspect pregnancy.

Anyone with a previous obstetric problem needs to discuss past events and may be offered treatment, where appropriate. For those couples with a genetic tendency to specific congenital abnormalities, such as Ashkenazi Jews (Tay-Sachs Disease), or those who have familial traits, genetic counselling should be sought.

References: CHAPTER 2

Department of Health (1992) "Women Advised to take folic acid to reduce risk of spina bifida babies" Department of Health Press Release H92/461 17 Dec

Hoffbrand A & Pettit J (1993) Essential Haematology 2nd Edition 1993 Blackwell Scientific Publications, London.

The Lancet editorial "Misconceptions about Preconceptual Care" The Lancet Vol.11, 9 Nov 1985 pp.1046-1047.

Lumley G & Astbury J Chapter 16 "Advice for Pregnancy" in: Effective Care in Pregnancy & Childbirth Eds: I Chalmers, M Enkins & M Keirse 1989 Oxford University Press, Oxford.

Rosenberg I H "Folic Acid and Neural-Tube Defects - Time for Action" New England Journal of Medicine 327 No.26 24 Dec 1992 pp.1875-1877.

CHAPTER 3

Diagnosis of Pregnancy

Many, and perhaps most, women know they are pregnant long before any test confirms it. There are certain early symptoms that can signal a pregnancy, for instance:

– change in food preferences
– increase in weight
– enlarged abdomen
– fatigue
– breast changes eg tingling/soreness (3-4 weeks), and changes such as enlargement, pigmentation of the primary and then the secondary areola, the dilatation of superficial veins and the presence of colostrum.
– nausea (4-14 weeks)
– amenorrhoea (4+ weeks)
– frequency of micturition (6-12 weeks)

Although none of these symptoms are definitive in themselves, they can suggest pregnancy to a suspicious woman. However, even without any definite signs, some women say they "just know".

"Quickening" is the term used to describe the first fetal movements felt by the mother, usually at about 18-20 weeks for a primigravida and about 16-18 weeks for a multigravid woman. Fetal movements are a positive sign of pregnancy.

CHEMICAL TESTS

Pregnancy testing kits can be easily purchased from any chemist by a woman wanting confirmation of her pregnancy. General Practitioners, Family Planning Clinics, and medical staff can also arrange for a test to be carried out.

Pregnancy testing has been available since 1928, when urine from women suspecting pregnancy was injected into immature mice. After four days the mice were sacrificed, and corpora lutea could be observed if sufficient human chorionic gonadatrophin (hCG) was present. Over the years rabbits and frogs were also used, but these biological tests have now been replaced by immunological tests.

HCG is still the basis for most pregnancy tests. When anti-hCG is added to urine together with latex particles or sensitized red cells, agglutination will only occur when no hCG is present.

The development of increasingly sensitive tests for hCG means that now tests can be made on urine with a dipstick coated with a specific monoclonal antibody to capture the antigen. This test can be carried out from the time of the first missed period when levels of hCG would be relatively low. (Redfern, 1985).

Proteinuria, or the presence of luteinizing hormone (caused, for instance by drugs such as some antipsychotics or some tranquilizers) can result in a false reading. (Taylor & Pernoll, 1987).

No pregnancy test is 100% accurate - false positives
and false negatives can occur, although most manufacturers claim at least 98% accuracy for their tests.

VAGINAL EXAMINATION
There are signs of pregnancy that can be noted on vaginal examination, but these are less commonly used now that chemical tests are so readily available and reliable.

Hegar's Sign (6-10 weeks)
This is rarely done as it has been suspected of causing abortion. One hand is placed behind the uterus abdominally and two fingers of the other hand are inserted into the anterior fornix of the vagina. Pregnancy softens the isthmus of the uterus to such an extent that the fingers of both hands almost meet.

Jacquemier's Sign (or Chadwicks's Sign)(8 weeks)
This is the change in colour of the vaginal membrane, to a bluish/purple, caused by the growth in vascularity of the vagina due to the increased oestrogen.

Osiander's Sign (8 weeks)

There is increased pulsation in the lateral vaginal fornices, due to the increase in vascularity associated with the enlargement of the uterine arteries.

Internal Ballottment (14 weeks)

With the fingers inserted in the vagina, on the cervix, a gentle tap upwards is made. The fetus moves away from the cervix and as it returns a tap is felt on the examining fingers.

ULTRASOUND

Pregnancy can be diagnosed very early by ultrasound scanning. At 5 weeks a fetal sac can be visualised, and the movement of the fetal heart and the small embryo can be seen at 6 weeks (Chamberlain et al, 1988).

Xrays should be avoided in early pregnancy because of the risk of damaging the developing fetus, (see Chapter 11) but if inadvertently taken, the fetal skeleton can be seen at about 14 weeks.

Definite confirmation of pregnancy can only be made:

- when the fetus can be palpated (about 22 weeks)
- when the fetal heart can be heard (about 10-12 weeks with a Sonicaid, and 24 weeks with a Pinard's stethoscope)
- by visualisation on ultrasound examination
- by visualisation on Xray.

References: CHAPTER 3

Chamberlain G, Gibbings C & Dewhurst J Illustrated Textbook of Obstetrics 1988 J B Lippincott Co., Philadelphia.

Redfern B "Pregnancy Tests" Mother Nov. 1985 pp.15-17.

Taylor C & Pernoll M Chapter 7 "Normal Pregnancy & Prenatal care" In: Current Obstetrics and Gynaecological Diagnosis and Treatment 1987 Eds: M Pernoll & R Benson 1987 Appleton & Lange, California.

CHAPTER 4

Blood Pressure Recording

Blood pressure is the pressure exerted by the blood on the walls of the blood vessels. It is determned by the following factors:

– pumping action of the heart;
– resistance to the flow of blood in the arterioles;
– elasticity of the walls of the main arteries;
– blood volume and extra cellular fluid movement;
– viscosity of the blood.

Two levels of blood pressure are recorded; the systolic pressure, which is the maximum pressure in the vessel during contraction of the ventricles; and the diastolic pressure, which is the pressure when the ventricles are at rest. The blood pressure is measured in the brachial artery using a sphygmomanometer.

It is certainly the most common screening test used, and is assessed from the very first antenatal visit to the final postnatal discharge check by the community midwife.

Considering what an important screening test blood pressure measurement is during pregnancy, standards of performance vary greatly. Although it is unlikely that any decision about a woman's care would be made on a single blood pressure reading, there is nevertheless a good argument that consistency between professionals could improve the care offered to women.

There have been specific recommendations made, by the British Hypertension Society, on recording blood pressure during pregnancy (de Swiet, l991a). These are:

– a large sphygmomanometer cuff should be used for any woman in which the bladder does not cover 80% of the arm circumference. Large cuffs should be used if there is any doubt, as errors are greater when using too small a cuff than with one too large.

- when assessing the diastolic pressure, K4 (Korotkoff sound 4 - the muffling of the beat) should be used in preference to K5 (the disappearance of the beat).

- women should be in a sitting position, or lying in the left lateral position, when having their blood pressure recorded, and the cuff should be approximately level with the heart.

The systolic reading is open to fewer differences of opinion than the diastolic pressure, and so would be a more convenient basis for treatment, but the diastolic has long been considered the more significant reading in pregnancy. However, the systolic reading is now beginning to be acknowledged as significant in predicting fetal outcome (de Swiet, 1991a).

A blood pressure recording is obtained as early in pregnancy as possible in order to determine a baseline measurement. Normal blood pressure measurements do change in pregnancy. Although there is only a small decrease of the systolic, the diastolic shows a marked fall due to progesterone relaxing the smooth muscle of the blood vessels and the reduced viscosity of the blood. It is at its lowest point in mid pregnancy, and then rises to the non-pregnant level at term (de Swiet, 1991b).

If the blood pressure reading early in pregnancy is elevated in a healthy woman she is said to have essential hypertension; - the cause of this is not generally known, but it is often found to be familial. If there is an identifiable cause for the hypertension, such as renal disease, it is known as secondary hypertension. A woman booking early in her pregnancy with a blood pressure of more than about 130/85mm/Hg would need close observation throughout her pregnancy, to ensure her condition does not worsen.

Women with either essential or secondary hypertension in a more severe form, with an initial blood pressure recording of more than 150/95 mm/Hg, may need anti-hypertensive medication started early in the pregnancy.

Pregnancy induced hypertension (PIH) usually does not manifest until the third trimester. The earlier it occurs, the more potentially serious the outcome.

Pregnancy induced hypertension is defined as a blood pressure recording of more than 140/90 mm/Hg, or a rise of more than 30 mm/Hg systolic and more than 15 mm/Hg diastolic above the first trimester booking blood pressure recording.

When pregnancy induced hypertension is associated with proteinuria (and sometimes oedema), it may also be known as pre-eclampsia. A woman with this condition must be carefully monitored, usually as an in-patient. The condition can worsen rapidly, especially in those early in the 3rd trimester, and put the life of both the mother and fetus at risk. The Report on Confidential Enquiries into Maternal Deaths in the UK covering 1988-1990 (Department of Health, 1994) lists hypertensive diseases of pregnancy as the most common cause of maternal death.

Nevertheless, it is true that most women who have mild pregnancy induced hypertension occurring in late pregnancy, usually have a good outcome. If there is a question of the baby's growth being compromised, or of the mother's condition deteriorating, then induction of labour is usually carried out. However, some studies have shown that the majority of cases of mild pregnancy induced hypertension in late pregnancy have been associated with larger than normal babies (Lancet editorial, 1991).

References: CHAPTER 4

Department of Health 1994 Report on Confidential Enquiries into Maternal Death in the UK 1988-1990. HMSO, London

Lancet - Editorial "Practice Imperfect" Lancet Vol.337, No.8751, 18 May 1991 pp.1195-1196.

de Swiet M "Conflicting Views on the Measurement of Blood Pressure in Pregnancy" British Journal of Obstetrics & Gynaecology Vol.98, No.3, March 1991(a) pp 239-240.

de Swiet M Chapter 18 in Scientific Foundation of Obstetrics and Gynaecology 1991(b) Eds: E Phillip & M Setchell 4th edition Butterworth/Heinemann

CHAPTER 5

Urine Tests

Urine tests were one of the first screening tests carried out by midwives. In the early 1900s midwives testing urine needed to heat specimens over spirit lamps (carefully boiling only half of the contents!) or add drops of various chemicals to diagnose 'pregnancy kidney' (Berkeley, 1924).

Most urine testing today is done quickly and accurately with reagent strips. Protein, glucose, ketones, blood, bilirubin and the pH of urine can be easily assessed. However, accuracy in using these strips is dependent on reading each component at the correct time - a procedure that it is only too easy to rush.

The colour, appearance and smell of the urine can also be significant, for example blood-stained appearance or a fishy smell. Most midwives make these observations automatically, only recording them in the case of an abnormality.

Proteinuria

In pregnancy urine is screened regularly, primarily for the presence of protein, which could indicate a urinary tract infection (very common in pregnancy) or could, when a rise in blood pressure has been noted, signify pregnancy-induced hypertension with proteinuria (see Chapter 4 for details). If protein is found in a clean mid stream urine(MSU) specimen, it should be sent for laboratory analysis to exclude infection, and the woman's blood pressure checked carefully.

In pregnancy-induced hypertension with proteinuria a 24 hour collection of urine is often analysed for protein. More than 500mg in 24 hours is considered to be a significant amount.

Glycosuria

Although glucose is an abnormal constituent of urine when a woman is not pregnant, in pregnancy it is a common feature and signifies a change in renal function rather than in carbohydrate metabolism. If glycosuria persists, serum screening for diabetes, such as a random blood sugar or a glucose tolerance test, if not already done, is carried out. (See Chapter 7 for details on serum screening for diabetes).

It is also worth considering that glycosuria is sometimes present with an infection. However, most women with glycosuria are just demonstrating the normal lowered renal threshold of pregnancy.

Ketonuria

Ketones are the by-products of a breakdown of fat and usually occur in either starvation or diabetes mellitus. If present, a woman may be suffering from, for example, distressing morning sickness, or her dietary intake may be erratic, and she will need appropriate advice. Diabetes should, of course, be excluded.

Blood

Blood is an abnormal constituent of urine and the woman needs to be questioned as to whether she has been bleeding vaginally (or perhaps rectally) and therefore has contaminated the specimen. The presence of blood in urine is most commonly due to a urinary tract infection, kidney damage (for instance associated with chronic renal disease) or systemic lupus erythematosus (SLE).

Creatinine Clearance Test

Creatinine is a naturally occurring metabolite and by measuring the amount passed in urine over a 24 hour period, renal function can be assessed (normally 1.2-1.7g). When a blood specimen is also analysed, the two values can determine the glomerular filtration rate (normal 90-110 ml/min but higher in pregnancy. This test is usually done as part of the assessment of a woman with pregnancy induced hypertension with proteinuriea.

Other tests

Metabolites of drugs injected can be analysed from urine specimens, and this may play a part in a reduction or detoxification programme for a drug misuser. Specimens should, of course, only be used for this purpose with the mother's permission.

Urinary oestriols and Human Placental Lactogen (HPL)

These tests have been used to assess fetal wellbeing in the past, although they have now been largely superceded by ultrasound where available. See Chapter 9 for further details.

References: CHAPTER 5

Berkeley C. A Handbook of Midwifery 6th Edition 1924 Cassell & Co. Ltd. London.

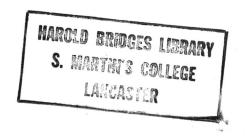

HAROLD BRIDGES LIBRARY
S. MARTIN'S COLLEGE
LANCASTER

CHAPTER 6

Weight Gain in Pregnancy

Weighing a woman at regular intervals during pregnancy is a traditional part of antenatal care. Most textbooks quote a recommended rate of weight gain for normal healthy women of about 2 kg up until 20 weeks gestation and 0.5 kg per week after that until term, with an average total weight gain of 12 kg. However, it is difficult to define what a normal weight gain is as women, and their attendants, have always been influenced by current theories about eating in pregnancy (which have varied greatly over the years) and in the past by superstition and folklore.

If a woman starts pregnancy at a normal weight for her height there seems to be an association between maternal weight gain and birth weight of her baby, but not a direct relationship (Altman & Hytten, 1989). One theory is that the rise in birth weight does not correlate with the increase in maternal body fat, but with maternal lean mass gain, and this depends much more on the woman's overall health and specific nutritional intake (Langhoff-Roos et al, 1987). Another suggestion is that the weight gain in the latter half of pregnancy is dependent on the level of oedema, which is a natural physiological response to pregnancy. Interestingly, even when associated with hypertension, studies show that those with oedema have heavier babies (Hytten, 1990).

Other than assessing fetal growth, the other reason most commonly given for the routine weighing of pregnant women is to detect pregnancy-induced hypertension. However studies show that the rate of weight gain is a poor predictor of pregnancy-induced hypertension, and blood pressure measurement and urinalysis continue to be the most reliable diagnostic tools (Dawes et al, 1992).

Women who are underweight before pregnancy have an increased risk of delivering a small-for-gestational age baby (Dawes & Grudzinskas, 1991). Those who are obese pre-pregnancy are more likely to have a large baby, and are also at increased risk of preterm delivery, pregnancy-induced hypertension and gestational diabetes (Narayansingh et al, 1988).

All women should be weighed at booking, and if their weight is within the normal range for their height, some would argue that no further routine weighing should be necessary (Hytten, 1990; Dawes et al, 1992). The time saved could be profitably used in monitoring those women who are under or over weight at booking and who may benefit from detailed nutritional counselling and closer observation.

However, others believe that it may still be of value to routinely weigh all pregnant women, and that this practice should not be abandoned without further research (Dimperio et al, 1992).

References: CHAPTER 6

Altman D & Hytten F Chapter 26: "Assessment of Fetal Size & Fetal Growth" in: Effective Care in Pregnancy & Childbirth Eds. I Chalmers, M Enkins & M Keirse 1989, Oxford University Press, Oxford.

Dawes M, Green J, & Ashurst H "Routine Weighing in Pregnancy" British Medical Journal Vol.304 No.6825 22 February 1992 pp.487-488

Dawes M & Grudzinskas J "Repeated Measurement of Maternal Weight during Pregnancy. Is this a useful practice?" British Journal of Obstetrics & Gynaecology Vol.98 No.2 February 1991 p.189

Dimperio D, Frentzen B & Cruz A "Routine Weighing during antenatal visits" British Medical Journal Vol.304 No.6825 22 February 1992 p.460

Hytten F "Is it important or even useful to measure weight gain in pregnancy?" Midwifery Vol.6, No.1 1990, pp 28-32.

Langhoff-Roos J, Lindmark G & Gebre-Medhin M "Maternal fat stores and fat accretion during pregnancy in relation to infant birthweight" British Journal of Obstetrics & Gynaecology Vol.94 No.12 December 1987 pp.1170-1177.

Narayansingh G, Rahaman J, Roopnarinesingh S "Obesity in Pregnancy" Journal of Obstetrics & Gynaecology Vol.8 No.4 April 1988 pp.307-309.

CHAPTER 7

Blood Tests in Pregnancy

Blood tests are performed frequently throughout the antenatal period, - most as a routine screening procedure, but some in response to developing symptoms manifested by the woman.

ROUTINE ANTENATAL BLOOD TESTS

Blood Group

(see Chapter 2 for a description of blood groups)

Rhesus Factor

The Rhesus factor takes on an importance during pregnancy because if a Rhesus negative woman has previously developed Rhesus antibodies, or develops them during the current pregnancy, there is a possibility of damage to any Rhesus positive baby she is carrying or may have in the future. If Rhesus antibodies are present in maternal serum, they can cross the placenta and affect any Rhesus positive fetus by causing haemolysis of fetal red cells. This can result in congenital anaemia, jaundice (mild or severe) or, if extreme, hydrops fetalis, a condition of severe oedema accompanied by enlargement of the liver and spleen which results in perinatal death.

For this reason all Rhesus negative women have blood tests to detect the presence of antibodies, usually three times during the pregnancy. If Rhesus antibodies are detected, they need to be quantified at regular intervals (at least every 2-3 weeks). If levels of anti D antibodies are less than 1 iu/ml (0.2 µg/ml) then no action is taken. If the level is 10 iu/ml (2.0 µg/ml), or rapidly rising, any Rhesus positive fetus is likely to be seriously affected (Hoffbrand & Pettit, 1993).

If antibody levels are rising, amniocentesis can be performed in order to assess the amount of bilirubin in the liquor, but there is a risk of a further feto-maternal transfusion. The amniotic fluid is scanned in a spectrophotometer for detection of bile products and the optical density can be measured. This provides an indication of the severeity of the disease. If the bilirubin level is rising dangerously, delivery will be expedited.

If the fetus is very immature, intrauterine blood transfusions may be required, but this, of course, is a hazardous procedure for the fetus. Rhesus negative blood of the same group as the mother is introduced into the fetal peritoneal cavity where it is absorbed by the lymphatic system within a few days. In severe cases the transfusion may have to be repeated on more than one occasion.

Other Antibodies

All antibodies are screened for in pregnancy as many of them may have an effect on the baby. (See Chapter 2 for details of potentially dangerous antibodies).

Full Blood Count

(See normal non pregnant values in Chapter 2)

During pregnancy plasma volume increases about 50% by 36 weeks and the red cell mass increases by about 18%. This extra circulating blood volume will obviously change the normal values of some haematological indices.

Haemoglobin (Hb)

Haemoglobin estimation is perhaps the most common of all antenatal blood tests. The fall in most women's haemoglobin during pregnancy, was previously taken by doctors as a pathological sign and all women were given iron tablets routinely on confirmation of their pregnancy. In fact this may still be appropriate in some parts of the world, where chronic anaemia contributes to the high maternal mortality.

The haemoglobin level is usually screened three times in pregnancy. The lowest acceptable reading seems to be 10g/dl although the World Health Organisation (WHO) cites 11g/dl. The lowest Haemoglobin should be expected at about 34 weeks when haemodilution has reached its peak.

It should be remembered that those woman who do not show signs of haemodilution may be at risk of developing complications in their pregnancy, in particular pregnancy-induced hypertension and small-for-gestational age (SGA) babies (Alexander et al, 1989). Some authorities believe that there is a possibility that giving iron supplements unnecessarily can raise haemoglobin levels artificially, so there is the same harmful effects as a lack of physiological haemodilution (Mongomery, 1990).

Mean Cell Volume (MCV)
The mean cell volume is the most sensitive index of iron status, as the earliest effect of iron deficiency is a reduced mean cell volume. The mean cell volume normally declines in early pregnancy and then rises in the second half, but the changes are small and within the normal non-pregnant range. Mean cell volume is also reduced with alpha and beta thalassaemia minor. A raised mean cell volume is associated with folate deficiency (high alcohol intake can reduce absorption of folic acid) or Bl2 deficiency.

Mean Cell Haemoglobin Concentration (MCHC)
Mean cell haemoglobin concentration falls in iron deficiency anaemia, but later than the mean cell volume.

Packed Cell Volume(PCV) Haematocrit
The packed cell volume falls in parallel with the red blood cell fall. In pregnancy the normal rate is 31%-34%.

Platelets
Platelets may progressively decline throughout pregnancy (especially after 32 weeks), but they usually stay within the normal non-pregnant range. Their function is related to coagulation and the clotting of blood.

As well as part of routine testing, platelets are also estimated in emergency situations, such as haemorrhage or intrauterine death, where the result can be used to help diagnose disseminated intravascular coagulation (DIC). In this condition there is widespread clotting in small blood vessels which affects the blood supply to various organs. Platelet levels will therefore fall.

White Cell Count(WCC) Leucocytes
Mean total white cell count is about 9.0 x 10^9/l. The total number of white cells rise in pregnancy, mainly due to the increase of neutrophils. During the first trimester, white blood cells number about 3000-15000/

mm^3, and in the second and third trimester about 6000-16000/mm^3. In labour white blood cells can rise to 20000-30000 mm^3. The state of pregnancy does seem to alter a woman's immunity somewhat with, for example, a decreased resistance in immune women to malaria, particularly during the first pregnancy (Cruikshank & Hayes, 1986).

Haemoglobinopathies

(See Chapter 2 for details of diagnosis pre-pregnancy.)

Woman are often first diagnosed as having thalassaemia minor or sickle cell trait from blood taken during their initial antenatal visit.

Electrophoresis testing can be carried out on blood samples taken from women identified as being at risk because of ethnic origin, or some laboratories test all blood samples with a reduced haemoglobin or mean cell volume.

The outcome of pregnancy in women with sickle cell disease has improved drastically over the past 15 years as a consequence of antibiotics, transfusion therapy and improved fetal surveillance (Lockwood & Hobbins, 1990).

However, these women are at risk of complications, especially if they already have organ damage, and this could worsen with increased sickling crises in pregnancy. Possible complications of pregnancy with sickle cell disease include miscarriage, urinary tract infection, pregnancy induced hypertension, preterm labour and intrauterine growth retardation. These women will need increased care in the antenatal period.

Alpha-Fetoprotein (AFP)

Alpha-fetoprotein is an alpha globin produced by the fetus and is present in the amniotic fluid and, in small amounts, in the maternal blood. The levels in maternal blood can be most accurately assessed between 16-18 weeks. Raised levels can indicate a multiple pregnancy, fetal death, an open neural tube defect in the fetus, wrong dates or just a false positive. Low levels can suggest a fetus with Down's Syndrome. (See Chapter 9 for further details.)

Triple Test

The triple test comprises testing of maternal blood for (i)alpha-fetoprotein, (ii)unconjugated oestriol and (iii)human chorionic gonadotrophin. These three levels, when considered with her age, will give the woman her degree of risk of carrying a Down's Syndrome fetus. (See Chapter 9 for further details.)

Blood Glucose Testing

Some form of diabetic screening is used in the majority of antenatal centres to diagnose gestational diabetes. Some centres may only test women who are deemed to be "at risk", such as those with a close relative who is diabetic, or those who have had a previous stillbirth or high birth weight baby. However, many centres now routinely screen all women antenatally.

Screening for gestational diabetes is most effective after 20 weeks of pregnancy, when the anti-insulin effect of the placental hormones is present.

Random Blood Glucose

A non diabetic pregnant woman's blood glucose is rarely above 5.5 mmol/l. A random blood glucose result of more than 7 mmol/l (or 7.7 mmol/l in some centres) would be an indication to investigate further for the presence of diabetes.

'Mini' Glucose Tolerance Test

An oral dose of 50g of glucose is given to a non-fasting woman, and blood is taken after 1 hour. A result of more than 7.7 mmol/l would be an indication for further investigations.

Glucose Tolerance Test

Glucose can be given orally or intravenously, although the most usual regime is 75g of oral glucose given after a fasting blood sample is taken. Thereafter blood is taken one, two and three hours later. The World Health Organisation defines a gestational diabetic as one whose fasting blood sugar is greater than 8 mmol/l, or whose 2 hour post 75g glucose load blood sugar is greater than 11 mmol/l. However, these values are disputed by many authorities, who prefer to calculate the various results to reach their own cut-off point.

4 or 6 Point Profile

A fasting blood sugar is taken in the morning and the woman then has blood taken immediately before (and after, in a 6 point profile) meals.

This will give a realistic picture of a woman's blood sugar levels, but it is an expensive test, as hospital admission for the day is usually necessary. Hospitalization is also inconvenient for the woman.

Glycosylated Haemoglobin A_1 (HbA$_1$)

The Glycosylated Haemoglobin A_1 test gives an indication of glucose levels over the preceding month. During pregnancy this test is usually carried out at every antenatal visit for all diabetic women. Non diabetic pregnant women usually score less than 8%, and this level should be the maximum for a diabetic pregnant woman, although many clinicians feel a lower rate would be more beneficial (Beard et al, 1987).

Infection Screening

Some infections are tested for routinely in the ante-natal period (for example, syphilis). See Chapter 8 for details on screening for infections in pregnancy.

ADDITONAL ANTENATAL BLOOD TESTS

Ferritin Levels (or Transferrin)

Ferritin levels are measured to identify the iron stores of a woman thought to have iron deficiency anaemia. The normal range is 15-300 µg/l. Serum iron fluctuates widely and is not a reliable indicator of iron status. Ferritin is a more stable guide and seems to be able to reflect iron stores accurately and quantitatively, particularly those in the lower ranges (Letsky, 1991)

Blood Clotting

Factors involved in the clotting mechanism alter during pregnancy. Fibrinogin levels rise almost 50% by the end of the second trimester to 400-500 mg/dl. Factors VII-X rise and factors XI + XIII fall.

Prothrombin (factor II) and factors V and XII remain unchanged.

These changes in the coagulation system in pregnancy occur in preparation for placental separation and the need to prevent haemorrhage from the placental site. However, together with increasing venous stasis in the legs during pregnancy, they can also predispose women to venous thrombosis. (Letsky, 1991).

Specific tests can be done to assess clotting ability. These are usually done in an emergency situation, such as haemorrhage or intrauterine death, or as part of an assessment of another suspected condition, such as deep vein thrombosis or pregnancy-induced hypertension with proteinuriea.

– Partial thromboplastin time (PTT) is the activated whole blood clotting time. This assesses the integrity of the intrinsic coagulation system. The normal range is 35-45 seconds.

– Prothrombin time (PT) measures the overall efficiency of the extrinsic clotting system. The normal range is 11-15 seconds.

– Thrombin time (TT) measures the final common pathway of the extrinsic and intrinsic coagulation system. The normal range is 10-15 seconds.

– Fibrinogin estimation tests are performed to determine the amount of functional fibrinogin present in the circulation. The normal range is 2-4 g/l.

Renal Function Tests

In pregnancy plasma creatinine falls, due to the normal dilution effect, the additional amount of blood circulating through the kidneys and the increased efficiency of the kidneys. The normal non-pregnant rate is 70-130 umol/l, but the upper limit in pregnancy would be 75 umol/l. However assessment of renal function in pregnancy should be based on creatinine clearance tests on 24 hour urine collections, as other factors can influence plasma creatinine results (Baylis & Davidson, 1991).

Plasma urea levels fall from a non pregnant rate of 2.5-5.8 mmol/l to 2.3-4.5 mmol/l in pregnancy because of altered tubal function.

The normal value for plasma urate is 0.15-0.42 mmol/l, but urate levels rise in pregnancies complicated by pre-eclampsia or intra-uterine growth retardation (Baylis & Davidson, 1991). In hypertensive women with a level of above 350 μmol/l (gestationally dependent), there can be significant perinatal mortality. An early sign of pre-eclampsia is a rising plasma urate, and this test is often done routinely when pregnancy-induced hypertension first manifests.

Renal function tests will be done, for example, for women with pregnancy induced hypertension with proteinuriea, renal infections such as pylonephritis, and for those with a history of renal disease.

Liver Function Tests

Normal non pregnant serum albumin levels are 40-50 g/l but they fall throughout pregnancy and at term are about 30% lower.

Normal non pregnant serum alkaline phosphatase levels are 35-105 iu/l, but by term these can increase two to four times. However, this is not a particularly relevant test of liver function during pregnancy, as the placenta also produces alkaline phosphatase.

Serum cholesterol levels (3.6-6.0 mmol/l in non pregnant women) can rise to about double at term.

In pregnancy serum bilirubin levels usually remain at the non-pregnant rate of 3.5-20.5 µmol/l.

Liver function tests are needed to diagnose particular liver disease such as Intrahepatic Cholestasis of Pregnancy, or Acute Fatty Liver Disease of Pregnancy. They are also done for any woman with a history of liver disease, and liver function tests are abnormal in many women with eclampsia.

Central Venous Pressure

Central venous pressure is the pressure of blood in the right atrium. It indicates the balance between cardiac output and venous return. Central venous pressures are unchanged in pregnancy, averaging about 10 cm H_2O in the third trimester.

Electrolytes

Electrolytes are substances which in solution dissociate into electrically charges particles (IONS). The concentration of electrolytes remain largely unchanged by pregnancy.

Table 3 Normal electrolyte levels

Sodium	135-145 mmol/l
Potassium	3.5-5.5 mmol/l
Calcium	2.2-2.6 mmol/l
Magnesium	0.8-1.3 mmol/l
Hydrogen Carbonate	24-28 mmol/l

Electrolye imbalance may occur in conditions such as severe vomiting or renal failure, and is diagnosed by examination of the serum.

Pre-eclampsia Profile

Most units use results of creatinine, urea and electrolyes, urate, liver function tests, platelets and clotting, plotted regularly on a graph, to give a complete picture of a woman suspected of pregnancy-induced hypertension with proteinuria. Results from twenty-four hour urine collections measured for protein and creatinine clearance would also be included.

References: CHAPTER 7

Alexander S, Stanwell-Smith R, Buekens P & Keirse M Chapter 29: "Biochemical Assessment of Fetal Wellbeing" in: Effective Care in Pregnancy and Childbirth Eds: I Chalmers, M Enkins & M Keirse 1989 Oxford University Press, Oxford.

Baylis C & Davidson J Chapter 11 "The Urinary System" in: Clinical Physiology in Obstetrics Eds: F Hytten & G Chamberlain Second Edition 1991 Blackwell Scientific Publications, Oxford.

Beard R, Hamilton-Fairley D and Elkeles R S "Problems & prospects for the pregnant diabetic" Modern Medicine December 1987

Cruikshank D & Hayes P Chapter 5 "Maternal Physiology in Pregnancy" In: Obstetrics - Normal & Problem Pregnancies Eds: S Gabbe, J Niebyl & J Simpson 1986 Churchill Livingstone, NY.

Hoffbrand A & Pettit J Essential Haematology Third Edition 1993 Blackwell Scientific Publications, London.

Letsky E Chapter 2 "The haematological system" in: Clinical Physiology in Obstetrics Eds: F Hytten and G Chamberlain Second Edition 1991 Blackwell Scientific Publications, Oxford.

Lockwood C J & Hobbins J C Chapter 1 "Haematologically mediated recurrent pregnancy wastage: identification and management of patients at risk" in: Hematologic Disorders in Maternal-Fetal Medicine Eds: M Bern & F Frigoletto 1990 Wiley-Liss Inc. NY.

Mongomery E "Iron levels in pregnancy, physiology or pathology? Assessing the need for supplements" Midwifery Vol.6 No.4 December 1990 pp.205-214

CHAPTER 8

Infection Screening

Women are, with exceptions, as immunocompetent during pregnancy as at other times, but some infectious diseases such as poliomyelitis, influenza or pneumococcal pneumonia may be more common (Stirrat, 1991).

While some infections are screened for routinely in all pregnant women, others are only tested for in those who have signs and symptoms. Most infections that are common in pregnant women are easily treated. The danger lies when the infection has crossed the placenta into the fetus, particularly during the first trimester of pregnancy because the fetus is at a vulnerable stage of development at that stage. The risk is compounded when the woman does not have, or does not recognize, symptoms and therefore does not seek treatment.

Infections can transfer to the fetus by three routes. Most viruses can cross the placenta and therefore pose a particular problem to the fetus as it develops. Infections can also ascend from the woman's genital tract in the presence of ruptured membranes, and during the actual birth process the baby can come into contact with maternal infection.

SCREENING BLOOD FOR INFECTION
Cytomegalovirus
Cytomegalovirus is a virus found in the salivary glands. It is the most common cause of intra-uterine infection, and although 50% of fetuses may be infected about 80% of them will develop normally (Griffiths, 1991). However, primary maternal cytomegalovirus infection can cause brain damage to the fetus during the first and second trimesters of pregnancy.

Other conditions which could occur in the baby include pneumonitis, neonatal hepatitis and various central nervous system disorders.

Cytomegalovirus can lay latent in maternal tissues and become reactivated during pregnancy (Stirrat, 1991). The presence of antibodies in the blood against cytomegalovirus is indicative of infection, and virus specific lgM antibody is present in acute infections (Farr, 1988). The virus may also be cultured from saliva and urine (Rowson et al, 1981).

Listeriosis

Listeriosis is caused by a gram negative bacteria found widely throughout the environment. It causes upper respiratory disease, septicaemia and encephalitic disease. Advice is given to pregnant women to specifically avoid soft cheeses, pâtes and to ensure cook-chill meals are well heated through. Symptoms may be mild or severe, and include malaise, headache, fever, backache and general influenza-like symptoms. Preterm labour or meningitis (of mother or baby) could result. Diagnosis is made by culture of blood or cerebrospinal fluid.

Hepatitus B

Hepatitus B is very common with more than 200 million carriers in the world. The virus is found in saliva, semen, vaginal fluids and blood. It is usually transmitted by injection of infected blood or blood products.

All women may be routinely tested at antenatal booking, or only women targeted 'at risk'. Risk categories include:

- – history of jaundice
- – blood transfusions/dialysis
- – injecting drug addicts
- – tattoos
- – a recent trip to a country with high levels of hepatitis.

Blood is screened for HbsAg and then tested for 'e' antigens. If a woman is 'e' antigen positive, then there is a greater risk of maternal/ fetal transmission and the baby will need treatment after birth (Griffiths, 1991).

Human Immunodeficiency Virus (HIV)

HIV is a retrovirus which is the causative organism of Acquired Immune Deficiency Syndrome (AIDS). It has been previously known as HTLV-III and LAV.

Support for the idea of offering the HIV test to all women at antenatal booking is increasing but it is questionable whether pregnancy is the ideal time for a woman to be tested (See Chapter 2). Anonymous testing is being carried out at many centres and contributes to statistics which monitor the growth of HIV in the heterosexual population. It must be remembered that even though the serum obtained for anonymous testing will not be marked with any identification, the woman must still give permission for her blood to be used.

All tests performed during pregnancy should be accompanied by some form of information sharing or counselling, but this is especially important for HIV. Counselling for this condition should be done by those who have undertaken formal training in counselling as well as having specialist knowledge of HIV.

The woman who tests positive will need much extra support, not only throughout her pregnancy, but probably for the rest of her life.

Two tests can be carried out - the ELISA test (Enzyme Linked Immunosorbent Assay) and the WESTERN BLOT TEST. If both are done the result should be at least 99% accurate.

An HIV positive woman may need extra tests during her pregnancy. Her T4 cell count will probably be estimated every 4-6 weeks: a level of 500-800 T4 cells means she is probably asymptomatic. Haemoglobin estimations may be done more frequently as there could be an increased risk of anaemia. Opportunistic infections are watched for carefully and prophylactic antibiotics may be prescribed.

Rubella

Rubella is a dangerous condition in pregnancy because the virus crosses the placenta to the fetus and may cause multiple defects and sometimes intra-uterine death. All pregnant women are tested for rubella immunity at antenatal booking. Some women who have been previously vaccinated, and, indeed, previously tested as immune, have been known to become infected, or tested as susceptible. There is obviously a strong case to be made for having rubella status checked prior to pregnancy (see Chapter 2 for details of pre-conception testing). Those women who are susceptible to rubella will be offered vaccination after their baby is born, but they will be at risk of contracting rubella during their current pregnancy. The new MMR (Measles, Mumps & Rubella) vaccine now offered to all young children should help to irradicate rubella in years to come.

Symptoms of rubella can include a macular rash on the body, a low grade pyrexia and a general feeling of malaise. These symptoms can be so mild as to be not noticed at all by the woman. If a woman reports a contact with rubella, or complains of the above symptoms, a blood test is done.

Since blood for rubella serology takes 17 days to produce rubella IgG antibodies, if these are present before 17 days she is probably immune. If retesting after 17 days shows no antibodies, this should be checked again 4 weeks after the contact.

If no antibodies are present, this should mean that there has been no infection (Griffiths, 1991). An infection can also be confirmed by the detection of rubella specific IgM antibodies, but these can show a false negative(Wang & Smaill, 1989).

Rubella can cause the loss of the pregnancy, or the birth of a rubella-infected baby with various physical and mental anomalies. These include cardiac, eye and ear defects and mental and physical retardation. The fetus is most vulnerable up until 16 weeks gestation, but the infection can cross the placenta at any gestation. An infected baby can be infectious for up to 2 years.

Syphilis

Syphilis, caused by the spirochaete treponema pallidum, is a sexually transmitted disease. It is rare in the UK but all women are screened antenatally because of the potential tragic effect on the fetus. Syphilis can cause loss of the pregnancy or the baby could be born with congenital syphilis, and may show signs of hepatosplenomegaly, anaemia, jaundice, snuffles and central nervous system involvement.

Most of the symptoms of syphilis such as the painless chancre in the primary stage, and non specific rashes and lymph node enlargement in the secondary stage, may easily go unnoticed.

Tests for syphilis include the treponema pallidum haemagglutination (TPHA), the rapid plasma reagin (RPR) and the venereal disease reference laboratory (VDRL).

The Wasserman reaction (WR) has been largely replaced by the VDRL test.

It is possible to get true positive test results with yaws and pinta, and false positive results with malaria, leprosy, tuberculosis and glandular fever (Hurley, 1991).

Syphilis is treated with antibiotics, penicillin G being the drug of choice. The longer the duration of the infection, the longer the course of treatment is necessary.

RPR or VDRL titres should be repeated monthly until delivery, and these serial blood tests should show a decrease in titres if the treatment is effective. VDRL titres are generally lower than RPR, therefore these tests should not be used interchangably when assessing the titre levels.

Toxoplasmosis

Toxoplasmosis is an infection caused by the parasite Toxoplasma gondii. It can be transmitted from domestic cat faeces, soil, raw meat and unpasteurised milk. The symptoms can be mild and influenza-like but most people have no symptoms at all. Infection can be confirmed by a rising titre (a positive titre of 1:500 or more is probably diagnostic), or the presence of specific IgM antibodies, but interpretation of serological tests can be difficult. Transmission to the fetus is less common, but more serious, during the first trimester(Wang & Smaill, 1989).

SCREENING VAGINAL DISCHARGE FOR INFECTION

Many women note an increase in vaginal discharge during pregnancy. If this is white or cream coloured, non-irritating and not offensive it is normal (physiological leucorrhoea).

Any discharge that is itchy or painful, offensive, or not a white/cream colour needs immediate investigation.

Candidiasis (Thrush)

Candidiasis is a fungal infection, usually candida albicans. It is common in pregnancy, especially in the third trimester and can affect any part of the body. The commonest sites are warm moist areas such as the vagina, mouth and skin folds(Shah, 1992). The diagnosis can be made on the clinical symptoms of itchy, sore red areas with white patches, but a swab should be taken to confirm the diagnosis by culture.

Candidiasis can be transferred from the mother to baby during birth, and the baby may manifest symptoms in his mouth or his buttocks. If a breast feeding baby has oral candidiasis, his mother's nipples should be checked, otherwise the baby may become reinfected after treatment, and the mother may continue to suffer sore nipples that could be cured. It is useful to check the woman's partner also, as he could be a source of re-infection.

Treatment for vaginal candidiasis (thrush) is usually by pessary or cream for local application, and clotrimazole, miconazole or nystatin are the anti-fungal drugs most often used. Oral thrush in the baby is usually treated with Nystatin drops.

Chlamydia

Chlamydia is a bacterial infection which is increasing rapidly in both men and women. Chlamydia trachomatis is usually asymptomatic in the woman but can be passed to the baby during birth. Infected babies can develop eye or respiratory infections (McGregor & French, 1991). Chlamydia can be diagnosed by culture of an endocervical specimen or by using antigen detection methods.

Genital Warts

The human papillomavirus (HPV) is the causative agent of genital warts, and their presence has been associated with genital cancers. The mode of transmission is usually sexual intercourse.

Genital warts are often treated with cytotoxic agents but these are contraindicated in pregnancy. Depending on the site, warts can be excised or removed by cyrocautery or electrocautery.

The warts may seem to disappear spontaneously but it is thought they can also reappear after treatment.

Since babies can develop laryngeal papilloma following a vaginal delivery by an infected mother, treatment of the warts should be done in the third trimester of pregnancy.

Gonorrhoea

Gonorrhoea is an infection by the gonococcus and is most usually sexually transmitted. Infected woman may have a purulent vaginal discharge or dysuria, but many women are asymptomatic.

The diagnosis is usually made by culture of a swab, although in acute infection direct examination of a gram-stained smear can be made. Since the gonococcus is susceptible to drying, swabs should be placed in transport medium (Hurley, 1991).

If left untreated in a woman, a gonococcal infection can ascend and become a cause of pelvic inflammatory disease. A baby born to a mother with gonorrhoea can contract gonococcal ophthalmia, typified by a copious purulent discharge from the eyes. This can cause blindness if not treated promptly.

For women, antibiotics, with penicillin as the preferred drug, is the treatment and is administered orally, intramuscularly or intravenously. The infected neonate is also treated with antibiotics, intramuscularly or intravenously and, in the case of gonococcal ophthalmia neonatorum, may also receive antibiotic eye drops.

Group B Streptococcus

Between 5-25% of pregnant women carry Group B streptococcus in their genital tract and suffer no ill effects. However this organism is the most frequent cause of sepsis in neonates, although the disease only occurs in 1-2% of colonized babies(Wang & Smaill, 1989). Treatment during pregnancy has not been shown to be effective, but intrapartum antibiotics have offered protection to the baby (Wang & Smaill, 1989).

Herpes Simplex

Genital herpes simplex is a virus that causes vesicular lesions, which can become latent and then reoccur, often at times of mental or physical stress (such as pregnancy). Although there is some evidence that the virus can be transmitted to the fetus via the placenta, it is thought that most cases of neonatal infection of the neonate are caused during the birth(Mercey & Mindel, 1991). Some women have cervical and vaginal viral swabs taken weekly from 36 weeks to diagnose a reoccurrence and, if a swab is positive, they are offered a caesarean section birth. Other women are assessed when in labour and a decision is made as to the mode of delivery then.

Trichomoniasis

Trichomoniasis is a sexually transmitted disease caused by Trichomonas vaginalis. It can be diagnosed by the symptoms of pruritis and painful vaginitis, and a change in vaginal discharge, sometimes to a frothy, greeny-yellow colour. A microscopic examination of a fresh specimen of the discharge, or culture, will diagnose the condition.

Urinary Tract Infection (UTI)

A urinary tract infection can be anything from a mild urethritis or cystitis to pyelonephritis. Symptoms usually include dysuria, frequency, renal pain and pyrexia. The most common causative organisms are Escherichia coli, proteus, faecalis, klebsiella and staphylococcus aureus.

Diagnosis of infection can be made on dipstick testing (blood and protein present) and laboratory testing quantitatively (100,000 organisms per ml signifies infection). Culture is necessary to identify the organism and sensitivity.

Untreated urinary tract infection may lead to preterm labour and permanent renal damage in the mother.

References: CHAPTER 8

Farr A Dictionary of Medical Laboratory Sciences 1988, Blackwell Scientific Publications.

Griffiths P D Chapter 50 "Virology" in: Scientific Foundations of Obstetrics and Gynaecology Eds: E Phillip & M Setchell 4th Edition 1991 Butterworth/Heinemann.

Hurley R Chapter 49 "Virology" in: Scientific Foundations of Obstetrics and Gynaecology Eds: E Phillip & M Setchell 4th Edition 1991 Butterworth/Heinemann.

McGregor J & French J "Chlamydia Trachomatis Infection during Pregnancy" American Journal of Obstetrics & Gynaecology Vol.164, No.16 suppl. June 1991, pp.1782-1789

Mercey D & Mindel A "Preventing Neonatal Herpes?" Genitourinary Medicine Vol.67, No.1, Feb 1991 pp1-2.

Rowson K, Rees T & Mahy B A Dictionary of Virology 1981, Blackwell Scientific Publications.

Shah P N "The Management of Candidal Infections in Pregnancy" Maternal and Child Health Vol.17, No.8, August 1992 pp 239,242-244.

Stirrat G Chapter IV "The Immunological System" in: Clinical Physiology in Obstetrics Eds: F Hytten & G Chamberlain 1991 Blackwell Scientific Publications, Oxford.

Wang E & Smaill F Chapter 34 "Infection in Pregnancy" in: Effective Care in Pregnancy & Childbirth Eds: I Chalmers, M Enkins & M Keirse 1989, Oxford University Press, Oxford.

CHAPTER 9

Tests for Fetal Diagnosis

HAROLD BRIDGES LIBRARY
S. MARTIN'S COLLEGE
LANCASTER

As tests to assess fetal well being and to diagnose abnormalities are becoming more commonplace, it is appropriate for midwives to remind themselves that these tests should never be routine. A midwife might suspect intrauterine growth retardation (IUGR) on abdominal examination and arrange for an ultrasound scan to assess the growth of the baby. She may be acting appropriately, but needs to be aware that labelling the baby as "not growing properly" might well be devastating to the expectant mother, who needs information conveyed to her in a sensitive manner.

No test should be done without adequate counselling with the parents. The more complex and life-changing the possible diagnosis might be, the more information and time the parents need before making their decision about whether to undergo the test or not. Parents need to know what is being tested for and exactly what a positive (and negative) result will mean, and give their permission for the test.

TESTS FOR GROWTH AND FETAL WELLBEING

Fetal Movements

The first fetal movements can usually be felt by a primigravida at 18-20 weeks, and by a multigravida at 16-18 weeks. Asking about the fetal movements is part of a midwife's antenatal check of a woman, but all midwives are aware that women can experience fetal activity differently - some are extremely aware of every movement and find them very uncomfortable, whereas others are barely aware of any movements. It is important to discuss fetal movements with a mother so that she becomes aware of her baby's pattern and realises the importance of reporting any deviations. A reduction or cessation of fetal movements can signal an impending stillbirth.

Many centres give women perceived to be 'at risk', or, in some cases, all women, 'kick charts' late in the third trimester of pregnancy. The

Cardiff 'count to ten' system is one of the most widely used. The woman contacts her midwife if she does not feel 10 distinct fetal movements in a set period of time (usually 12 hours).

Fetal Growth

Fetal growth is assessed at every antenatal visit by means of measuring the fundal height against maternal anatomical landmarks and/or measuring the fundal height to the symphysis pubis with a tape measure. Some studies have proved the latter a successful method of detecting intra-uterine growth retarded (IUGR) babies, especially when there is continuity of the clinician, but other studies have found it less successful (Altman & Hytten, 1989). Where ultrasound is available it is often used to confirm, or rule out, fetal growth retardation (see Chapter 10 for more information on the uses of ultrasound). It must be remembered that although small for gestational age is usually defined as a weight under the 10th centile, most of these babies will be perfectly healthy and normal.

Biochemical Assessments

Biochemical tests include assays of oestrogens in maternal blood or urine and formerly, human placental lactogen in maternal serum. Because of their poor predictive powers, biochemical tests have largely been replaced by biophysical studies in the UK (Alexander et al, 1989). However, in some parts of the world these tests are still in use.

Oestrogen Screening

Oestriols form 90% of the total oestrogens found in pregnancy and, since the placenta produces oestriol in conjunction with the fetus, oestriol measurement has been seen as an assessment of placental/ fetal wellbeing,

The assessment of oestriols can be made from a 24 hour urine collection or a serum specimen, the latter being considered more reliable. A low level of oestriol excretion can be associated with fetal intrauterine growth retardation and before the advent of biophysical profiles a falling level on serial estimations in late pregnancy was considered an indication for intervention.

Cardiotocography (CTG)

Continuous fetal heart monitoring for periods of about 30-60 minutes may be carried out in high risk women to assess the condition of the fetus. There have not been any randomized controlled trials that have demonstrated a benefit from routine cardiotocography (CTG) monitoring during pregnancy (Wheeler, 1991). Nevertheless, it can be reassuring to the clinician, as a normal cardiotocography trace can indicate a well oxygenated fetus at the time of the test in 99% of cases. However, an abnormal cardiotocography trace will probably only indicate hypoxia in 14% of cases (Murphy et al, 1990).

Interpretation of a cardiotocography trace involves:

– baseline fetal heart rate: normally 120-160 beats per minute(bpm) although 110 to 120 can be considered normal in a term baby if all other aspects are satisfactory.

– variability: the variation in the baseline rate over 1 minute. The normal value is 5-15 bpm. Periods of poor variability ('sleeping trace') are usually about 20-30 min. An unexplained 'sleep' trace of more than 40 minutes can be a sinister sign.

– accelerations (reactivity): a temporary rise in the baseline of more than 15 bpm for 15 seconds or longer. This is usually in response to fetal or maternal movement and is regarded as a sign of fetal well-being. The normal value is at least 2 accelerations per 15-20 minutes.

– decelerations: a slowing of the fetal heart from the baseline of at least 15 bpm for at least 15 seconds. Decelerations are divided into:
• early (synchronous with a contraction and amplitude less than 40 bpm),
• late (the peak of the contraction and the lowest part of the deceleration have a lag time of more than 15 seconds), or
• variable (described as an early deceleration with an amplitude greater than 40 bpm, or variable in shape and occurring at variable times during contractions).
Decelerations unprovoked by contractions are a worrying sign.

(Steer, undated)

Although interpretation of a cardiotocography trace may appear straightforward, a trace can sometimes be very difficult to decipher and research has shown that it can vary from one clinician to another (Mohide & Keirse, 1989).

BIOPHYSICAL PROFILE

A biophysical profile is a combination of assesments by ultrasound and cardiotocography, which is used to assess the wellbeing of the fetus. The biophysical variables include:

– fetal breathing movements
– gross body movements
– fetal tone
– qualitative measurement of amniotic fluid
– reactive fetal heart rate

Each of these variables is assessed and a numerical value is usually attached to the findings. The observation of normal fetal movements, tone and heart rate, and at least one pocket of fluid measuring >1 cm in two perpendicular planes, will score '2' for each variable, totalling '10' - a fetus that could be defined at low risk for chronic asphyxia. Any abnormal observation would score '0', and a low total score may lead an obstetrician to suspect chronic asphyxia and consider immediate delivery. (Gabbe, 1986).

The biophysical profile is concerned with detecting the 'at risk' fetus, but because of its high cost, it is commonly used as a diagnostic, rather than a screening test.

Doppler Ultrasound

Doppler ultrasound is used to investigate utero-placental and fetal blood flow. It records the fetal heart pulsations and indentifies blood velocity waveforms in the fetal umbilical artery. It is thought that alterations in the fetal umbilical blood flow may occur in early fetal compromise.

DIAGNOSTIC TESTS

Alpha-fetoprotein (AFP)

(See Chapter 7 for a description)

Serum alpha-fetoprotein levels can be assessed in the mother's blood at 16-18 weeks. This is the time in pregnancy when the test is most reliable. The level will be elevated in most pregnancies in which the fetus has a neural tube defect. It can also be elevated for other reasons such as wrong dates, multiple pregnancy, threatened abortion, intra-uterine death or other anomalies (Turner's syndrome or omphalocele for example).

A major disadvantage of the test is the many false positives - it is estimated that for every 25 women having a single elevated alpha-fetoprotein level, only 1 will eventually prove to have a child with a neural tube defect (Simpson, 1986). For this reason women with a single elevated result should have a repeat test. If this is also elevated a detailed anomaly scan and, perhaps, an amniocentesis should be performed. Liquor alpha-fetoprotein is a more accurate test than serum alpha-fetoprotein.

A low alpha-fetoprotein level can indicate Trisomy 21 (Down's Syndrome). See triple test for further information.

Chorionic Villus Sampling

A small biopsy can be taken from the developing chorion, via the cervix or trans-abdominally, at 9-12 weeks, which can be analysed for fetal chromosomal abnormalities in a few days. This has been seen as a great advantage over amniocentesis, as the results would probably be available in time for a first trimester termination if that was appropriate. However, the miscarriage rate following chorionic villus sampling is higher than after amniocentesis. This could be because the rate of spontaneous miscarriage at this time is much greater than that later in pregnancy. Also recent studies have indicated there may be some link between chorionic villus sampling and limb abnormalities (Lilford, 1991).

Amniocentesis

Amniocentesis is usually carried out from 15-16 weeks under ultrasound and strict aseptic conditions. A needle is inserted through the abdominal wall into the uterus and about 20 ml of amniotic fluid is withdrawn. There are usually a few viable cells in the fluid that can be cultured, and in about 2-3 weeks these will have grown enough to analyse the chromosomes.

The timing of the diagnosis, necessitating a late termination if appropriate, is a big disadvantage of this test. There is a risk of about 1% of a miscarriage following the procedure, and a chance of infection if strict asepsis is not observed. A Rhesus negative mother should always be given anti-D immunoglobulin following any invasive procedure, to prevent Rhesus isoimmunisation.

Early amniocentesis is practised widely in the USA and is becoming more common in the UK. In American studies, looking at amniocentesis done at or before 12 weeks, there seems to be a higher miscarriage rate compared with those done later than 15 weeks, but this is perhaps not the fault of the procedure as spontaneous abortion is more common earlier in pregnancy. There is also the possibility of missing an abnormality that would be diagnosed if tested later. However, the women have the undoubted advantage of an early diagnosis. (Hanson et al, 1992).

Since the risk of carrying a baby with Down's Syndrome (the most common chromosomal abnormality) is increased with age, in the UK most women over 35 are offered amniocentesis.

Beside fetal karyotyping, more than 60 different inborn errors of metabolism can be diagnosed using amniotic fluid (Fisk & Rodeck, 1989).

Amniocentesis can also be carried out to confirm the diagnosis of neural tube defects after a positive serum alpha-fetoprotein result, although this is rarely done as diagnosis can usually be made by ultrasound.

Fetal pulmonary maturity can be assessed by testing the amniotic fluid for the lecithin:sphingomyelin ratio. A lecithin-sphingomyelin ratio of 2:1 indicates adequate surfactant in the fetal lungs and therefore respiratory distress syndrome of the newborn is unlikely to occur. This test is rarely done, as the risk of amniocentesis is unacceptable now the fetus can be assessed by biophysical means, and the prognosis of preterm babies is so improved.

Triple Test

The triple test consists of the results of serum alpha-fetoprotein, serum unconjugated oestriol and serum human chorionic gonadotrophin (hCG), taken together with the mother's age, to calculate the risk factor of a fetus with Down's Syndrome. This is done at 16 weeks gestation, and since the normal serum values of human chorionic gonadotrophin, alpha-fetoprotein and oestriols vary with gestational age, it is extremely important to have accurate dates.

As the result is only a risk calculation, not a diagnosis, the woman must then decide whether to have an amniocentesis for a specific diagnosis. The actual odds of those with a positive screening test being affected is 1 in 43 (Wald et al, 1992).

Triple Test Plus

This is the triple test, as described, above with the addition of urea resistant neutrophil alkaline phosphotase (NAP). It is not yet performed routinely as more information is needed to correlate the results with the other substances screened, and the test is not yet automated. However, measurement of urea resistant neutrophil alkaline phosphotase may be the most accurate marker to detect Down's Syndrome in the future. (Cuckle et al, 1990).

Fetoscopy

An instrument called a fetoscope is inserted into the uterus transabdominally. Examination of the fetus under direct vision can be done from about 15 weeks, to diagnose structural abnormalities and to obtain skin, tissue and blood samples (see fetal blood sampling). Fetal blood transfusions can also be given if necessary when Rhesus isoimmunisation has occurred.

Fetal Blood Sampling (FBS)

Fetal blood sampling can be carried out under direct vision by fetoscopy or under ultrasound (cordocentesis). The usual site sampled is the umbilical vein about 1 cm from the placental cord insertion. Blood obtained can be used to diagnose many conditions such as haemoglobinopathies, chromosomal abnormalities and congenital infections. Assessment of the fetal blood for signs of haemolysis or chronic hypoxia can also be made. There is a risk of miscarriage of about 2-5% following cordocentesis and also a risk of maternal haemorrhage or infection (Daker & Borrow, 1989).

DNA Probes

At present DNA testing is not common, but it is the area that shows the most potential for the future. As experience and knowledge in using this technique grows it will be possible to diagnose most abnormal fetal conditions, and even identify those which may be carriers (Weatherall, 1991).

References: CHAPTER 9

Alexander S, Stanwell-Smith R, Buekens P & Keirse M Chapter 29 "Biochemical Assessment of Fetal Wellbeing" in: Effective Care in Pregnancy Eds: I Chalmers, M Enkins & M Keirse 1989 Oxford University Press, Oxford.

Altman D & F Hytten Chapter 26 "Assessment of Fetal Size and Fetal Growth" in: Effective Care in Pregnancy & Childbirth Eds: I

Chalmers, M Enkins, & M Keirse 1989 Oxford University Press, Oxford.

Cuckle H, Wald N, Goodburn S, Sneddon J, Amess J & Dunn S. "Measurement of activity of urea resistant neutrophil alkaline phosphatase as an antenatal screening test for Down's syndrome" British Medical Journal Vol. 301   3 November 1990 pp.1024-1026.

Daker M & Borrow M Chapter 23 "Screening for genetic disease and fetal anomoly during pregnancy" in: Effective Care in Pregnancy & Childbirth Eds: I Chalmers, M Enkin & M Keirse. 1989 Oxford University Press, Oxford.

Fisk N & Rodeck C Chapter 9 "Antenatal Diagnostic Procedures" in: Fetal Monitoring Ed: J Spenser 1989 Castle House Publications Ltd. Kent.

Gabbe S Chapter 10 "Antepartum Fetal Evaluation". in: Obstetrics - Normal & Problem Pregnancies Eds: S Gabbe, J Niebyl & J Simpson1986 Churchill Livingstone, NY.

Hanson F, Tennant F, Hune S & Brookhyser K "Early amniocentesis: outcome, risks and technical problems at <12.8 weeks" American Journal of Obstetrics & Gynaecology Vol. 166 June 1992 pp.1707-11.

Lilford R J "The Rise and Fall of Chorionic Villus Sampling" British Medical Journal Vol.303 No.6808 19 October 1991

Mohide P & Keirse M Chapter 30 "Biophysical Assessment of Fetal Wellbeing" in: Effective Care in Pregnancy & Childbirth. Eds: I Chalmers, M Enkins, M Keirse. 1989 Oxford University Press, Oxford.

Murphy K et al "Birth Asphyxia and the Intrapartum Cardiotocograph" British Journal of Obstetrics & Gynaecology Vol.97, No.6 June 1990 pp470-479.

Simpson J L Chapter 8 "Genetic Counselling & Prenatal Diagnosis" in: Obstetrics - Normal & Problem Pregnancies Eds: S Gabbe, J Niebyl & J Simpson 1986 Churchill Livingstone, NY.

Steer P J Fetal Heart Monitoring: Surgicraft Pocket Guide (undated) Surgicraft Ltd., Reddrich.

Wald N, Kennard A & Densem J "Antenatal Maternal Serum Screening for Down's Syndrome: Results of a Demonstration Project" British Medical Journal Vol.305, No.6850, 15 August 1992 pp.391-394.

Weatherall D J The New Genetics and Clinical Practice 3rd edition 1991 Oxford University Press, Oxford.

Wheeler T Chapter 53 "Cardiotocography" in: Scientific Foundations of Obstetrics and Gynaecology Eds: E Phillip & M Setchell 4th edition 1991 Butterworth/Heinemann.

CHAPTER 10

Ultrasound Scans

Ultrasound is high frequency, low-intensity sound waves which can be 'beamed' into the body via a transducer. "Echoes" from the different surfaces within the body are reflected back to produce a two-dimensional picture on a screen in shades of grey. As the transducer is moved over the abdomen, different views (vertical, oblique or transverse) can be shown (Fisher & Russell, 1975). Since air acts as a barrier between the body and the transducer, a special oil or gel needs to be put on the abdomen.

HISTORY

There has been no research done to properly evaluate the safety of ultrasound, although it is a routine part of antenatal care in the UK today. Some studies done in the USA have suggested the possibility of a higher incidence of dyslexia, and, more recently, research conducted in Norway indicates an increased incidence of left-handedness in children who had been scanned in utero. There is also a large study from Australia showing the possibility of smaller babies following increased scanning in pregnancy (Newnham et al, 1993). However, there is so far no clear evidence that the use of ultrasound in human pregnancies has any harmful biological or physical effect (Neilson & Grant, 1989; Keirse, 1993).

Nevertheless, many women today are anxious about the lack of clearcut evidence of safety, and the fact that their fetus may be submitted to lengthy exposure to ultrasound during the antenatal and intrapartum period. The amount of exposure experienced by a fetus can vary immensely according not only to the number of ultrasound scans performed, but also the type of equipment used and the duration of the examination (Gabbe, 1986).

The Association for Improvement of Maternity Services (AIMS) are now providing women with a form on which to record these variables and other ultrasound exposure (eg sonicaid, electronic fetal heart monitoring) as they believe these details should be part of every woman's and baby's health record (Association of Improvement in the Maternity Services, 1993).

As well as abdominal scanning, vaginal ultrasound is now possible using a special probe. This is particularly useful up to 12 weeks gestation to obtain a better picture and aid earlier diagnosis. It also avoids the discomfort experienced by the woman of being scanned with a full bladder, as is necessary for abdominal scans in early pregnancy (Kenyon, 1989). However, those who are concerned about possible side effects of ultrasound argue that vaginal scans expose the fetus to more ultrasound at a vulnerable time, and that there is not the protection that maternal tissue and amniotic fluid offer when abdominal ultrasound is used (Association of Improvement in the Maternity Services, 1993).

USES OF ULTRASOUND

Diagnosis of Pregnancy

(See Chapter 3 for details of diagnosis of pregnancy with ultrasound.)

Estimation of gestational age by ultrasound

During the first trimester measurements taken of the fetus can usually date the pregnancy accurately to within 5 days. In the second trimester accurate dating is possible to within 1-2 weeks. Fetal measurements, however, are not useful in assessing gestational age after 30 weeks. A routine dating scan can mean a reduced number of inductions for presumed post maturity (Neilson & Grant, 1989). It can also be useful when tests (such as alpha-fetoprotein or the triple test) are carried out, as an accurate result can depend on correct dates.

Fetal Investigations

Ultrasound is valuable in visualising the fetus and placental site when carrying out invasive investigations or treatment of the fetus such as amniocentesis or fetal blood transfusion.

Anomaly Screening

Anomaly scans are offered in most centres at 16-22 weeks. This appears to be becoming more a routine examination rather than a procedure about which women make an informed choice. It is of course the midwife's responsibility to ensure all women have enough information to consent to, or refuse, an anomaly scan when it is offered.

In an anomoly scan, fetal anatomy is examined and many structural abnormalities can be diagnosed. New anatomical pointers for various conditions are frequently being discovered as operators become more experienced and equipment more sophisticated. Examples are the suggestion that the presence of a black 'space' behind the fetal neck could be indicative of Down's Syndrome, or that measurements of the fetal ear could predict abnormality.

Accuracy of anomaly scans vary, and it is unlikely anywhere can offer 100% accuracy. This refers not only to missed conditions, but also to 'false positives' where fetuses are diagnosed with an abnormality they do not have.

Multiple Pregnancy

Multiple pregnancies can be easily diagnosed by ultrasound. By 5-7 weeks twins gestation can be visualised as two completely separate sacs.

Placental Siting

When routine scanning is done at 16-20 weeks, it is often noted that the placenta is lying low in the uterine cavity. However, as the uterus grows the placenta 'moves up' and only a small proportion of these women will have a placenta previa. Ultrasound is not 100% accurate in identifying placenta previa, even in late pregnancy, as it is particularly difficult to identify the lower segment when the placenta is posterior.

Assessment of Fetal Growth/Well-Being

Measurements of the fetus can be used to determine whether its growth is sufficient, or suboptimal. It will usually be necessary to undertake serial scans to get a full picture. If the fetus's abdominal circumference growth is slow, or indeed reducing, in comparison with the biparietal diameter measurements, then this could identify an 'at risk' fetus where intervention was indicated. Likewise a baby can be diagnosed as exceptionally large, which would alert the care givers to the need for careful observation in labour and delivery.

Observation of the fetus's activity, as well as environment, can form part of other tests (for example, biophysical profile or doppler ultrasound - see Chapter 9) to assess the well being of the fetus.

Malpresentations/Malpositions

Ultrasound can identify presentations and positions that could make successful labour difficult (or impossible). The information it provides can help determine the mode of delivery.

Placental Grading

Some studies have identified the physiological changes in the placenta, and suggest that early maturation can be associated with fetal complications in labour (Proud, 1989).

ADVANTAGES AND DISADVANTAGES OF ULTRASOUND

Ultrasound is now part of routine antenatal care. It has obvious advantages, such as early detection of some serious anomalies, giving women sufficient time for a termination if that is their wish. Women do see ultrasound as an instrument that can reduce their anxiety, but even repeated scans cannot guarantee a woman a perfect baby.

When treatable conditions are diagnosed antenatally, then the delivery can be planned for an appropriate place and time. Certain conditions, such as some obstructions of the renal system, can now even be treated in utero. However, the news of even a minor anomaly can alter the parents' outlook and affect pre-natal bonding as the parents may focus on the abnormality rather than on the growing baby.

References: CHAPTER 10

Association for Improvement in the Maternity Services AIMS Quarterly Journal Vol.5 No.1 p.17 Spring 1993. Fisher A & Russell J Radiography in Obstetrics 1975 Butterworths

Gabbe S Chapter 10 "Antepartum Fetal Assessment" in: Obstetrics: Normal & Problem Pregnancies Eds: S Gabbe, J Niebyl & J Simpson 1986, Churchill Livingstone, NY.

Keirse M "Frequent prenatal ultrasound: time to think again" The Lancet Vol.342 9th October 1993, pp.878-879.

Kenyon S "Making Sense of Obstetric Ultrasound" Nursing Times Vol.85 No.31 2 August 1989 pp 39-41.

Neilson J & Grant A Chapter 27 "Ultrasound in Pregnancy" in: Effective Care in Pregnancy & Childbirth Eds: I Chalmers, M Enkins & M Keirse 1989, Oxford University Press, Oxford.

Newnham J, Evans S, Michael C, Stanley F & Landau L "Effects of frequent ultrasound during pregnancy: a randomised controlled trial" The Lancet Vol.342 9 October 1993 pp.887-891

Proud J Chapter 5 "Placental Grading" in: Midwives, Research & Childbirth Vol.1 Eds: S Robinson & A Thomson 1989 Chapman & Hall, London.

CHAPTER 11

Xray

The role of Xray in obstetrics has diminished drastically, as ultrasound has taken over many of its previous functions. Additionally, the dangers of Xrays to the fetus have become well known.

The fetus can be damaged by Xray exposure in several ways. Studies have shown a rise in the cancer rate, especially leukaemia, in those fetuses who were subjected to Xrays. There is also the chance of damage to the developing structures of the fetus, especially if the Xray is taken during the early organogenesis period. Damage can be caused to the reproductive cells of the fetus which could lead to abnormalities in the next generation (Fisher & Russell, 1975).

In the past Xrays were used for placental siting, but a particularly large dose of ionizing radiation is needed for this investigation. Xrays were also used to 'date' pregnancies in the third trimester, and this was done by looking at the bone age of the fetus, especially the developing centres of ossification of the knee and ankle. However, these functions, together with that of diagnosing multiple pregnancies, are now carried out by ultrasound.

If it is necessary for a pregnant woman to have a chest Xray, the best time is between 14-24 weeks, after organogenesis and before the uterus pushes the diaphragm upwards, causing compression of the lower lobes of the lungs.

Xray pelvimetry may still be performed, especially postnatally, to assess the size and shape of the bony pelvis after a caesarian section delivery carried out for suspected cephalopelvic disproportion. Pelvimetry will provide information for the next pregnancy. The resulting measurements, however, are often inconclusive (Krishnamurthy et al, 1991).

In the antenatal period a pelvimetry is sometimes carried out on a woman with a breech presentation, to help the obstetrician recommend the safest mode of delivery. However, even with accurate pelvic measurements, it is difficult to anticipate how the pelvis will accommodate the passage of the baby in labour, as the size alters not only under the influence of progesterone softening the ligaments, but also with the woman's posture.

Xrays can confirm fetal death, by showing gas in the heart and large blood vessels of the fetus, and by identifying the collapse of the skull and malalignment of the vault's bones (Spalding's sign)(Fisher & Russell, 1975).

References: CHAPTER 11

Fisher A & Russell J Radiography in Obsetetrics 1975 Butterworths

Krishnamurthy S, Fairlie F, Cameron A, Walker J & Mackenzie J. "The role of postnatal xray pelvimetry after Caesarean section in the management of subsequent delivery" British Journal of Obstetrics and Gynaecology Vol.98 No.7, July 1991 PP.716-718.

CHAPTER 12

Clinical Pelvic Assessment/Vaginal Examinations

In the absence of chemical tests, or ultrasound, early pregnancy can be diagnosed, and dates estimated, by obtaining a history from the woman and making a physical examination (see Chapter 3).

Vaginal examinations can be carried out during pregnancy, although many clinicians (and women) prefer to avoid them. There is no documented evidence that a routine vaginal examination will cause a miscarriage, but should a woman subsequently spontaneously abort, she may well blame the procedure. As with all examinations and tests, the procedure should only be done with the woman's consent, and all findings need to be carefully recorded.

One reason for a vaginal examination in the antenatal period is to perform a cervical smear for a previously unscreened woman.

Cervical Smears

Cervical smears, also called Papanicolaou smears, were developed in the 1940s by Dr Papanicolaou. There are now widespread cervical screening programmes for carcinoma throughout the UK.

Grading of smear tests and CIN (cervical intra-epithelial neoplasia) grade is as follows:

SMEAR	CLASS	CIN
I	Normal cells	-
II	Atypical cells	-
IIIA	Mild dysplasia	1
III	Moderate dysplasia	2
IV	Severe, carcinoma in situ	3
V	Invasive carcinoma	

Classes I and II are non-malignant but, class II cells have a change that may signify a viral or other infection. Class III is suspicious and may need either a repeat smear in 3 months or a biopsy. Classes IV and V are positive and require biopsy (Royle & Walsh, 1992). Biopsy is necessary to confirm the diagnosis of carcinoma, as a smear test only reveals abnormal (dyskaryotic) cells.

Infection

During pregnancy signs and symptoms of a genital infection may need to be investigated by speculum examination and a vaginal swab would be necessary to provide a diagnosis.

Pelvic Assessment

A vaginal examination can be carried out late in pregnancy to assess the size and shape of the pelvis and the risk of cephelo-pelvic disproportion.

The obstetrical conjugate is the measurement from the sacral promontory to the posterior border of the symphysis pubis. It is the diameter the fetal skull has to negotiate to enter the pelvis.

This cannot be measured accurately on vaginal examination but it can be estimated by attempting to reach the sacral promontory and noting where on the examining hand the lower border of the symphysis pubis reaches. This measurement (the diagonal conjugate), less 2 cm, is an estimation of the obstetrical conjugate. If the sacral promontory cannot be reached, the size of the pelvic brim is likely to be adequate.

Although it cannot be measured, the pelvic cavity can be assessed by noting the curve of the sacrum and the depth of the sacrosiatic notch - two fingers should fit easily into this. The outlet is assessed by noting the prominence and relative closeness of the ischial spines and estimating the angle of the pubic arch, which should be about 90°.

After the vaginal examination, the distance between the ischial tuberosities can be assessed by placing a closed fist on the perineum, where it should fit comfortably between them.

Although a pelvic assessment in late pregnancy can give a rough idea of the size of the pelvis, the outcome of labour is dependent on many other factors. A decision on the mode of delivery is unlikely to be made on the evidence of the pelvic assessment alone.

References: CHAPTER 12

Royle J A & Walsh M Watsons Medical-Surgical Nursing & Related Physiology 4th Edition 1992 Bailiere Tindall, London.

CHAPTER 13

Ethical Issues Surrounding Antenatal Testing

Antenatal tests which identify easily treatable conditions and can improve the well-being of mother and child are usually non-controversial. However, much screening, especially in the area of fetal diagnosis, provides many ethical dilemmas.

As more tests become increasingly widely available, mothers may not feel comfortable with their pregnancies until the fetus has been certified "normal". There is evidence that this is already happening with anomaly scans, which are now often a routine procedure. There is no way now, nor in the foreseeable future that medical science can guarantee a healthy baby. However, waiting for blood results which only give a risk score, having scan findings checked for various anomalies, or waiting for an amniocentesis and then the results, can place a very great stress on the pregnant woman, and a stressful pregnancy is known to be associated with poor obstetric outcome (Sandall, 1992).

On the other hand, if the technology is there, surely women are entitled to have fetal diagnosis and the option to terminate the pregnancy. Antenatal investigations, if the results are negative, can reassure not only the mother, but also her care-givers. Tests such as biophysical profiles have probably reduced the number of unnecessary interventions. Also, there are fetal diagnoses that can be made that will guide the place, mode and timing of delivery to the benefit of the baby and mother. In addition, some conditions are diagnosed that can be treated in the antenatal period.

It could be argued that antenatal screening and treatment of the fetus can be very expensive, and has an unsure outcome, but this is the on-going problem of who decides what cost is put on preserving a life - a debate which is as old as medicine, and probably will continue as long as medical treatment exists.

New techniques, especially DNA testing, are going to raise more ethical problems. When most diseases can be diagnosed antenatally, who will decide which conditions should or could be terminated? In theory the parents, as now, should of course make that decision - but what if they decide they do not want a child with a relatively minor disorder, such as an enzyme deficiency? Will the doctor feel obligated to terminate a fetus which he/she knows has the potential of a happy and fulfilled life?

Already some women are feeling the pressure of society's disapproval if they choose not to have antenatal screening, or termination of pregnancy when a fetal abnormality is diagnosed. Mothers aged over 35 who refuse antenatal investigations and have a Down's syndrome child could be regarded as having chosen this "burden on society" by default. As testing and diagnoses become even more sophisticated, will all mothers feel this obligation to only produce a "perfect" child? Society seems to have moved from an acceptance that some babies will be born handicapped, to the idea that women will abort those fetuses which are abnormal. This movement could well continue to encompass the idea that all "abnormality" is unacceptable.

Paradoxically, just at a time when there is a greatly increased ability to diagnose fetal abnormality, with the assumption of accompanying termination of pregnancy, there is also a growing anti-abortion movement in society.

Increased antenatal testing is also going to raise other difficult situations for individuals. When not only disease, but also carrier states can be diagnosed, are these individuals going to be stigmatised?

There is also the problem of what to do with information that will not be relevant for some time. At present, for example, those who have a family history of Huntington's Disease may well seek diagnosis before they have children, in order to plan their life. Others in the family would find the knowledge that they will become distressingly ill in middle age too much to bear and choose not to seek early diagnosis. If a condition in the fetus is diagnosed which manifests itself in later life, who then decides whether that child/adult should know, and when? This can be carried further, as evidence grows of a gene-link propensity to early heart disease. If this is diagnosed in fetal life, it could be argued that this child could avoid all adverse conditions that could contribute to cardiovascular problems. However, if this tendency to heart disease was known, how would that influence his future employment, or insurance, prospects?

The midwife has a great influence over the mother's experience of antenatal care. It is important that all midwives reflect on all the issues that arise, as only by being fully aware of her own feelings and attitudes, will she be able to offer the women as close to unbiased and non-judgmental care as possible.

References: CHAPTER 13

Sandall J "Prenatal Screening for Down's Syndrome" MIDIRS Midwifery Digest Vol.2 No.1 March 1992 pp.37-39.

Index